"When I Learned to Breathe"

Living with Asthma and 29 Allergies

By Leon L Welch

Introduction

I wrote this book as an inspiration to others "like me," who suffer with asthma, allergies or anything similar to what I have experienced. I'm here to serve notice that these ailments do not have to be roadblocks to reaching future goals!   I was embarrassed during my childhood when my friends found out I suffered with asthma.   I was treated different, bullied and felt inferior.   There were many things I wanted to do but couldn't such as take gym as a child, run long distance or swim, etc.   I feel indebted to my parents for taking care of me growing up because, it was not easy.   Even now, experiencing chest tightness, sinus congestions and ear infections, have been constant reminders of my past struggles. I recently found out I had 29 allergies!   Yet, with the support of my Doctor, family and friends, I learned to breathe! Nothing can stand in my way from achieving my goals in all aspects of my life!   I hope that this book is put to good use as an integral part of someone's plan to learn how to breathe.

Foreword

When Leon Welch told me he was writing a book, I had no doubt...he WOULD write a book. There is nothing that Leon doesn't do that he puts his mind to! I have worked with Leon for over four years. I have never known him to give less than 110%; whether as a diet technician, personal trainer, father, and friend. He carries with him strength in the Lord and a song in his step. He is motivating. He is motivated. His personal experiences continue to inspire others by the life he leads and example he sets. He is a true role model for youths and anyone who wants to overcome adversity and succeed.

Several years ago, as the Registered Dietitian for the long term care facility where both Leon and I worked, I was overseeing a weight loss challenge. While Leon certainly did not NEED to lose weight, he was motivated to achieve a goal and win. Leon was tied for 1st place with another employee, but he desperately wanted to win the entire prize. So, almost tongue in cheek, I said, "You need to burn 3,500 calories a day to win." Sure enough, the next day Leon brought me a picture of the exercise equipment he used and right there on the calories burned screen was "3,500 calories". It took him nearly 4 hours to do it! And he continued that for the next week or so and ended

up winning the whole jackpot!
Whether you suffer from asthma, or any struggle in life, this book shows you the proof of positive attitude and resilience. I hope you find Leon's words a source of comfort and inspiration for whatever you are trying to achieve.

With warmest regard,
Stefanie Jarrett, RDLD
Registered Dietitian

Table of Contents

Chapters

CHAPTER 1

Elbows and Knees

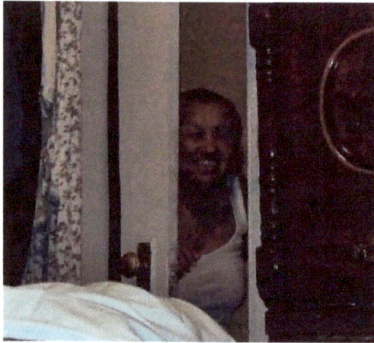

Sleeping was not easy to do as a child.   I tossed and turned most of the night.   I snored which disturbed my brothers while I tried to sleep lying on my back.   I coughed and wheezed loud enough that my back and head would hurt badly.   My deepest breath was like sipping through a straw.   I cried myself to sleep many nights!   One day in the middle of the night, I grabbed my pillow and tucked it between my elbows and knees.   I was in this position because it gave me comfort during the middle of the night after waking up due to having difficulty breathing.   My behind was now in the air as I slept all night on my elbows and knees. My Mom, bless her heart, would open the door to check on me and there I was balled up with my pillow, sleeping on my elbows and knees. I was sleeping like a baby. Did this stunt my growth? I'm unsure. All I wanted to get was a good night sleep!

CHAPTER 2

No Gym!

My gym teacher and I could not see Eye to Eye! Well, he was very tall for one and here I was this little kid that kept looking upward to him saying, "I can't take gym!" My favorite slogan, "I'm sick." Finally, after missing days of school and not having my gym clothes when I did come to gym class the gym teacher stated, "You need a Doctor's excuse or else you will not be excused from taking gym in my class." WOW! This was serious I thought! "I'm telling my mother," was the thought that was running through my mind!

Low and behold, my Mom got my excuse from the Doctor and I took it to gym class. The gym teacher saw me once again not dressed for gym. I walked up to him with this precious piece of paper and handed it to him. He gave me the meanest look I ever wanted to see and said, "Ok, you are excused, you can sit on the bench." "Really," I thought, I've been doing this all along! My life as an elementary kid changed. All my classmates and friends found out why I missed so many days of school and why I could not participate in gym class. I no longer felt normal. A new life begins with my public announcement of my illness.

CHAPTER 3

"Away with the liquid medicine"

My classmates always looked out for me in elementary. I would hear one of them say, "He can't play with us or he will get sick." I would think to myself, "thanks for the broadcast." I missed many days of sunshine watching my brothers and neighbors play from the inside window of my house! My Dad, bless his heart, would take me outside, stand me on the driveway to get some air and then I would come back in the house. Many times during the day I would sleep on the couch. I guess I was making up for sleep I missed through the night. Also, I smelled like Vick's © Vapor Rub throughout my childhood because I caught colds a lot and it helped ease my cough.

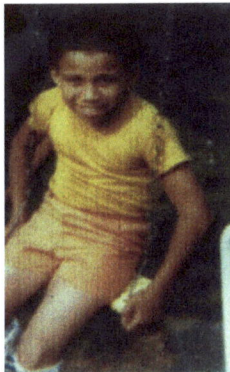

Junior High came and along with it, a new Doctor.   This Doctor took me off my liquid medicine and prescribed me an inhaler.   I had to carry this thing in my pocket all the time!   I didn't want the kids to see me with it or they would tease me. I did a good job hiding it!   I also was able to take gym, thanks to my new sidekick, my yellow inhaler. My breathing was restored to normal quicker than me using the liquid medicine I was use to taking.   What a break through!   I was able to play outside with my brothers and friends.   Vicks © Vapor Rub still hung around though because I still caught colds. When I caught a cold, breathing was very difficult.   When it was cool outdoors, my Mom always told me to put a hat on and zip up my coat before I got sick. Guess what? I got sick.   I didn't participate in any sports while in Junior High because of my asthma.   I was just beginning to learn "how to breathe."

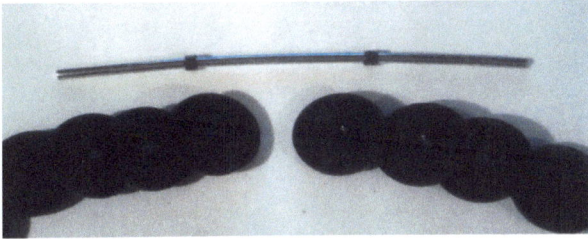

Chapter 4

The Bar!

Here I am in the ninth grade. I was not only battling asthma, I was the shortest kid in the school! The high school kids thought a parent left their child behind because I was so small in stature. I was given a growth shot, but it didn't help. I was bullied constantly. Some kids in my neighborhood also picked on me because others did. My homeroom teacher took me under his wing because we looked alike, felt bad for me and he was "vertically challenged" himself.

Tenth grade arrived and my Dad told me to come to the basement, I did. What do you know; my Dad had got a weight set! I looked at him intently like, "What in the world is this!" Nonetheless, he showed me what to do with the weight set and went along his way. My brothers began to work out and so did others in the neighborhood. I realized that I didn't have trouble breathing after lifting with the weight bar so I began to work out too. One day at a neighbor's house, all the kids were lifting weights. I was the last to participate since I was the smallest and weakest. When everyone was finished working out, all the weights were stripped and only the bar was left. The bar was heavy enough for me to get a good workout. However, everyone went outside and left me to train alone. "I'll get stronger," I said to myself, "they'll see."

CHAPTER 5

Finally, a Sport I Can Participate In!

I kept lifting with the bar and I got a little stronger. I began to add small weights to the bar. It's the beginning of summer! I'm done with tenth grade. I kept lifting with no trouble breathing unless I had a cold or flu. After working out for the whole summer, I was lifting all the weights (about 110 lbs.) in the basement. We had those old plastic cement weights and I religiously worked out the way my Dad showed me. At the beginning of my junior year in High School, all my friends noticed that my body changed. I put on muscle!

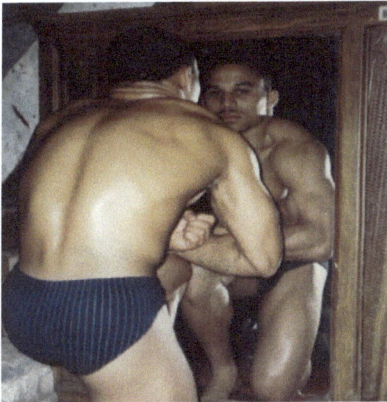

"Preparing for competition"

One day a friend told me, "You should get on the weight lifting team, my friend is on it." I simply said, "Okay." So, he took me to his friend's house. When I arrived, I discovered we shared a mutual friend from elementary school. I also discovered this guy had cast iron weights, he wasn't playing!" To my surprise, I was able to bench press 135 pounds. This was a decent feat for a guy who weighed roughly 115-120 pounds (with a cement suit on). "Not bad for a start, I'm going to introduce you to the weight lifting coach,"stated my friend.

The following day, we went to school and walked into the weightlifting coach's class. Low and behold, it was my homeroom teacher from ninth grade, the one who took me under his wing to protect me from bullies. "If you're serious, we will work out on Saturdays at my house," the coach said. The first Saturday at his house changed the rest of my life. I am finally able to participate in a sport without having difficulty breathing.

CHAPTER 6

Setting Records

At my coach house, I went to work getting prepared for my first ever sports competition. I told my Mom I was going to win a medal or trophy and she said, "You can do whatever you put your mind to Leon." My Dad, is one of those "Doubting Thomas" kind of guys—a real "I have to see it to believe it," person. I qualified for the weight lifting team and my weight class was between 100-120 pounds. I had no problem making weight for this weight class. Naturally, I was a small guy anyway. It seems like the disadvantages and weaknesses I perceived I had when I was younger became my strengths!

I competed at my first ever weightlifting competition and placed second. I was so happy to bring a trophy and medal home that I almost ran the entire way without worries about my asthma! My parents were proud and my Brothers too. My coach told me, "good job!" "Next year, were going to break records!" I thought to myself, "I'm lucky next year if I win first place!" I began training the beginning of summer before starting my senior year in high school.

At this point, I was well in control of my asthma. I enjoyed working out because I finally received positive attention from my peers. In fact, I no longer had bullies, because the people, who scared me in the ninth grade, now feared that I could beat them to a pulp! I was no longer the weakest kid in school and definitely not in the neighborhoods' basement gym. All the kids who left me in the basement to train alone flocked around me looking for tips to improve. I longed for the days when I trained alone. Improving me for competition was my only priority! My coach told me what to do and I did it. The two major lifts were the bench press and dead lift. I spent more time bench pressing though. I also noticed a major problem. Heavy weight training caused me to put on 15-20 pounds of muscle since my junior competition.

My coach did not care! He said, "I want you to compete in the 100-120 lb. weight class. You will have no problems and I believe you will set a new record." I reluctantly agreed and I understood how hard it would be to lose weight and keep strong. My Mom bought me a snow suit to jog in so I can keep warm outside during the fall-winter season. I got everyone's attention, but not for the right reason. The snow suit was peach in color! Well, fully embarrassed, I jogged at my old elementary school playing field near my house. Everything changed though! Instead of listening to jeers and jokes, I was cheered on as if I was Rocky Balboa getting ready for a boxing match.

After training, my coach (bless his heart,) entered me into a men's pause bench press competition at a local YMCA. I weighed more than 120 pounds, more like 132 pounds. I placed second. Good job for a first time teenager competing with men. In this event, I had to lower the bar to my chest and wait till the judge said lift. I ended off with a pause bench of 270 pounds. I won another trophy and my parents were again proud. Next, my high school competition! Asthma well under control, I was a neighborhood celebrity. Some neighborhood kids went to different high schools and they told me that I was the talk of the upcoming weight lifting competition. I weighed 135 lbs. and I was bench pressing 300 lbs. However, I was preparing to dominate the 100-120 lb. weight class. I had to lose weight! Living in a peach snow suit and weight loss behind me; the records for my 100-120 lb. weight class were:

Bench Press: 185 pounds

Dead Lift: Between 400-480 pounds.

The competitors at the competition already knew who I was. There were five representatives from my high school team while other schools had way more. In my weight class, my competitor ended the last of his 3 attempts on the weight bench at 225 pounds.

The coach said "See, you have no competition!   I want you to start off your first attempt at 225 pounds."   I simply said, "Ok." My bench press attempts went like this; first 225 lbs., second 240 lbs. and final 250 lbs.

My final dead lift attempt was 360 lbs.   I did it!   I set a new Bench Press record of 240 lbs. and a Total Lift record of 600 pounds in the 100-120 lb. weigh class.   My coach and team mates were proud. Our school placed third as a team.   Nothing felt better than hearing my name on the speaker in my homeroom during the morning school announcements of my achievements. I graduated from high school with trophies, medals, respect and a new friend.

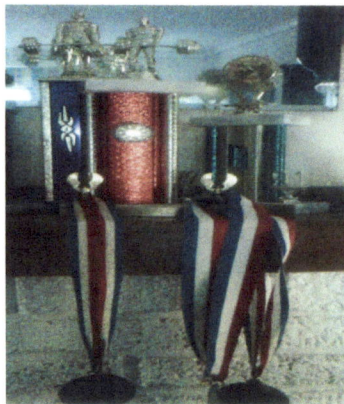

"My trophies and medals"

CHAPTER 7

From Homeroom Teacher, to Coach, to my Friend!

If it wasn't for my coach's belief in me, I never would have broken and set records in weight lifting. He told me I reminded him of himself when he was my age. I use to horse play with one of my friends during workouts at my coach house and he would yell down the stairs, "Let's get serious." My coach treated me like gold! He never talked about my asthma. As a matter of fact, nobody did anymore! He encouraged me to continue power lifting in competitions and maybe body building.

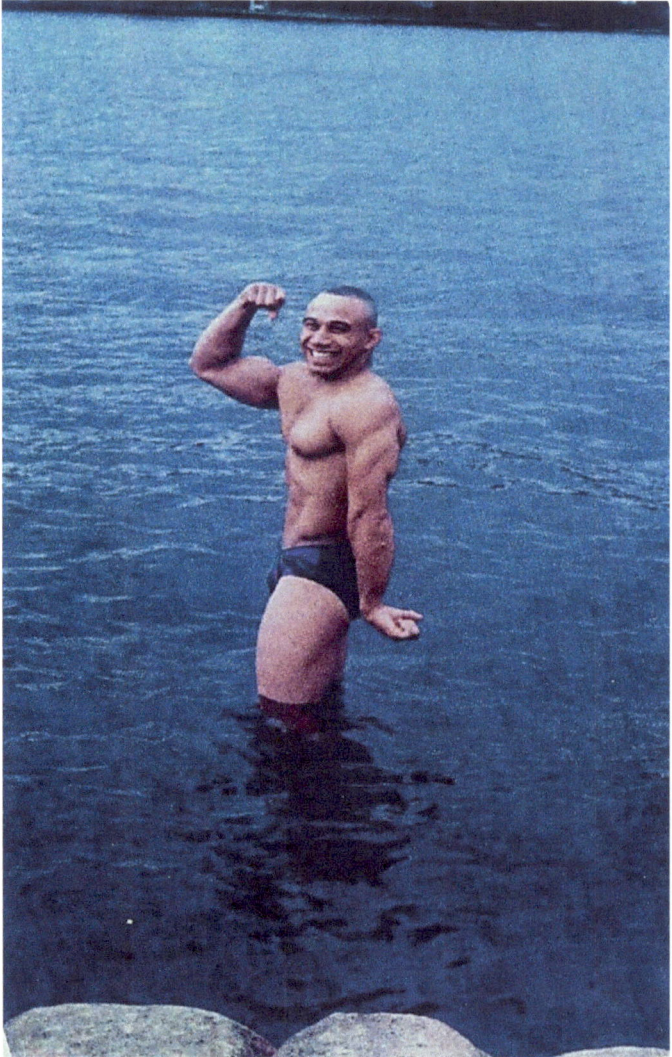

"Photo taken in Georgia, I weighed 140 pounds."

He treated me with respect.   I am today who I am when it comes to exercise due to his belief in me to rise above many obstacles I faced in life.   To go over and beyond in anything I wanted to do! He taught me the true meaning of God blessing a person to do exceedingly and abundantly above all you could ask or think!   He will always live on through my life.

CHAPTER 8

29 Allergies

Fast forward, I am around 32 years of age. I still get sick beyond the average person. I cut grass, breathe dust, run in cold or hot air, go into a house with pets and I would notice within an hour, I can't breathe. I scheduled to take an allergy test out of curiosity. My Mom told me I took one as a child. I never knew the results of it or even if I was prescribed medication. The Doctor told me, "Do not scratch your arms after you are pronged and shake them up and down." I thought, "ok, what is about to happen?" I had all these ink marks placed on both arms, 15 an arm. Then, I was injected with their test. My arms flared up very red! I was itching so bad that I wanted to cut my arms off! After my arms slowly stop itching, the Doctor came in and said, "I never seen anyone with this many allergies! You are allergic to 29 out of 30 allergies. You should live in a bubble!"

Patient name: Leon Welch Date of birth: 7/1/72

General information about skin test protocol

1. Location: back___ forearm___ Device: Hollister-Stier ComforTen / Quintest
2. Intradermal: 0.02 ml injected, Location: arm Testing concentration: 1:1000 w/v or 200 BAU or AU/ml
3. Results: Longest diameter of wheal (W) and flare (F) measured in millimeters at 15 minutes
   Scoring: 1+ = F < nickel (21mm), 2+ = F > nickel (21mm) + wheal <3mm
   3+ = F + wheal > 3mm , 4+ = F + wheal with pseudopods

Allergen:	Percutaneous W/F	Percutaneous Score	Intradermal W/F	Intradermal Score	Allergen:	Percutaneous W/F	Percutaneous Score	Intradermal W/F	Intradermal Score
INDOOR ALLERGENS (A)	X	X	X	X	**WEEDS/MOLDS (B)**	X	X	X	X
1. Cat hair			XXX	XXX	31. Kochia/burning bush				
2. Cat yolk			XXX	XXX	32. Rough pigweed				
3. Dog hair/dander					33. Short ragweed			MIX	MIX
4. Cockroach mix					34. Giant ragweed				
5. Aspergillus fumigatus					35. Cocklebur				
6. Dust mite farinae					36. English plantain				
7. Dust mite pteronyssinus					37. Dock/sorrel mix				
8. Penicillium notatum					38. Lamb's quarters				
9. Histamine control					39. Trichoderma (mold)				
10. Saline control					40. Stemphyllum (mold)				
GRASSES/TREES (C)	X	X	X	X	**MOLDS (D)**	X	X	X	X
11. Bermuda grass			XXX	XXX	41. Alternaria tenuis				
12. Johnson grass			XXX	XXX	42. Hormodendrum cladospor				
13. Kentucky blue grass			XXX	XXX	43. Phoma herbarum				
14. Orchard grass			XXX	XXX	44. Mucor racemosus				
15. Red top grass			XXX	XXX	45. Fusarium vasinfectum				
16. Rye grass			XXX	XXX	46. Epicoccum nigrum				
17. Timothy grass			XXX	XXX	47. Helminthosporium				
18. Beech (tree)					48. Pullularia pullulans				
19. Red mulberry (tree)					49. Curvularia spicifera				
20. Red cedar (tree)					50. Rhizopus nigricans	← not allergic			
TREE ALLERGENS (E)	X	X	X	X	**OTHER INHALANTS (F)**	X	X	X	X
21. American elm					51. Horse hair/dander				
22. Pecan/Hickory					52. Guinea pig hair/dander				
23. Cottonwood					53. Gerbil epithelia				
24. Eastern oak mix					54. Hamster epithelia				
25. Box elder/maple					55. Mouse epithelia				
26. Sycamore					56. Rat epithelia				
27. Black walnut					57. Rabbit epithelia				
28. White ash					58. Parakeet feathers				
29. Black willow					59. Candida albicans (mold)				
30. Birch mix						X	X	X	X

"Allergy test I took in Ohio".

I'm glad he thought it was funny! This explains why I constantly got sick. Also, I get motion sickness, ear and sinus infections to add to my wonderful list. Anytime I heavily sweep, cut grass, play with dogs and cats, stand around in cold or hot weather, exist on Earth, I get sick. Once I got sick, it took a long time to get my breathing back to

26 | P a g e

normal. Everything highlighted on my allergy test in pink, I am allergic to.

Basically, I have to take an allergy pill for life! I refuse to take allergy shots. I'm surprised as a child I survived! My allergies seem invincible in my life along with asthma, which makes breathing (even today) very difficult for me. I still remember after high school being invited by a good friend to an Air Force recruitment meeting. I impressed my friend's Air Force Representative with my physique until he asked me if I was on any prescribed medications. I told him, "yes!" Let's just say that made me in eligible for a desk job in the Air Force! Even worst, I lost out on a job opportunity at an ink factory because I failed the breathing test!

I had a lumber yard job and I did not know how bad I was hurting myself by being exposed to extreme changes in weather and tons of dust. Jobs were not easy to get. One winter day, at the lumber yard, I was not feeling well and that didn't matter, I had a line full of customers! My medicine was low in my inhaler. I had breathing difficulty beyond my usual and my inhaler ran out. I was rushed to the hospital! At the hospital, I was on my elbows and knees on the floor (a familiar childhood comfort position!)

I had to wait an hour before I was seen. A Doctor finally took care of me. I immediately received two breathing treatments. I was given some prescriptions and I left. When I got to the drug store, my breathing began to go haywire! I had to wait for my prescriptions to be refilled on my elbows and knees. Unfortunately, the Pharmacist told me (30 minutes later) my prescriptions could not be filled. I drove home, took off my lumber yard snow suit and crawled up the stairs. I was on my elbow and knees with my pillow tucked under me (a familiar childhood comfort position.)

My breathing patterns were short and I was aching all over. I thought, "This is it, I'm going to die!" What am I going to do? I'm alone! My Mom was away somewhere and my Dad was at work." My phone rang. Thankfully, it's my Brother! With all the strength I could muster up I said, "I can't breathe do you have your inhaler?" My Brother stated, "I'm on the other side of town, call 911."

Disappointed, I just hung up the phone and told myself, "This is it, I'm going to die!" I was in excruciating pain. I just laid there thinking about how long it would take for me to die. How long will I suffer? How long does it take for you to die from your lungs closing up! Well, obviously God wasn't through with me yet! Within minutes, (that felt like hours,) my Brother showed up and gave me his inhaler. You really cherish every breath you take when you only have a few left! Moments later, my Mom came home and stated, "Why are you so pale?" I told her, "Ma, it's a long story!" After this episode, I learned that I had to avoid outdoor jobs at all cost!

CHAPTER 9

Compassion for others

I am thankful for my parents, family, Doctor, friends and coach. They played a huge role in helping me learn how to breathe. I have a passion to help others because people showed me compassion. When I learned to breathe, I enjoyed doing things that I couldn't do before. I trained very hard for these goals. I was able to run a mile without passing out, swim an entire pool underwater, squat over 500 lbs., dunk a basketball on a regulation height basketball rim with the help of someone throwing the ball to me, jump over a car vertically and most of all continue to exercise safely and help others learn how to breathe in their time of need.

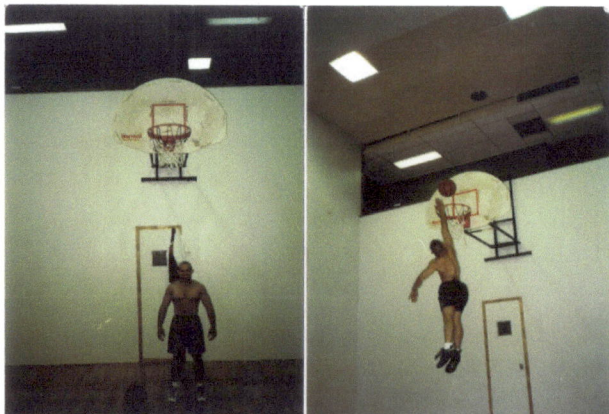

"After hours of training my legs, found out I could dunk on a 10 foot regulation rim."

After high school, I had many neighborhood kids grow up and workout with me. This one kid always came to the side door of my parent's house, knocked on my door and asked, "Can I work out with you?" I really did not take him serious. I mean, he was a short little pudgy kid that didn't look like he could lift a grape! However, he reminded me of someone I knew all too well, me! I began showing this kid everything I knew! Well, he grew up, played high school football and later went on to college. I was ecstatic I was able to pay it forward. I always wondered what he was doing.

In October of 2010, we ran into each other at his uncle's house. He asked me, "Can you help me? I need your help really bad!" Boy, this sounds familiar! I did not take him serious again! I told him that I will work with him two days a week. Well, it has been over 2 years now that we've been working out together. Wait, it's probably better if he tells his story of how I helped him learn how to breathe. A childhood friend of mine and workout buddy Jerome Peterson Jr.!

Chapter 10

Jerome Peterson's Story

There are a couple times in my life that made me change my outlook on life. Most recently, May 5th, 2009; but I'll get to that later. One of my first life-altering moments happened in the late 80's (I was nine years of age) when I met this guy name Leon Welch. He was vertically challenged (5 feet 1 inch tall) and from a distance, he didn't seem like much! Nonetheless, he would easily change your mind when you saw him back-flipping down the street for about 50 yards non-stop. Actually, I thought he was amazing!

Growing up in the inner-city, we didn't get to go to the circus (or any other event for that matter,) so watching this guy perform acrobatics was the highlight of my day! It was also very inspiring because I was a state-of-the-art wimpy fat kid who was also vertically challenged. However, I wanted to be healthy!

My family has a history of diabetes, high blood pressure, congestive heart failure, etc. I knew that it was important for me to stay healthy. I just didn't know how! He always invited the neighborhood kids to his house for weight-lifting, so maybe he would let me join! "You too little, Rome!" Sadly, that's what he told me.   I wouldn't give up!   I destined to work out with Leon.

Years passed and I was now in tenth grade! I wanted to play football. I was still that state-of-the-art wimpy kid!   So, I went back over Leon's house and asked him, "Can you help me workout?" I saw the look of reluctance in his face, but he relented. He gave me a fool proof workout system that allowed me to lose weight two months ahead of schedule and right before football practice started.

This new found strength and conditioning was amazing!   The principles he taught me allowed me to successfully compete in football and live a healthy lifestyle. I really got into running and before I realized, I was running 8 miles per day; 4 days a week. I remained healthy and vibrant all the way into my late 20's, when something seemed to change for the worst.

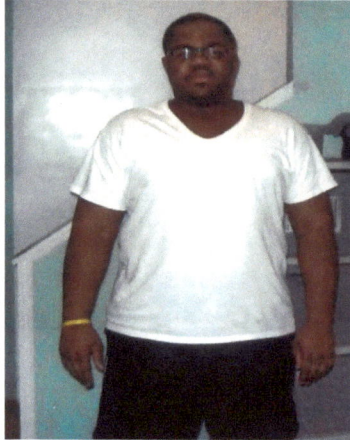

"First day of training with Leon"

CHAPTER 11

MCD and I don't mean McDonald's

In my late 20's, I was still following the principles Leon showed me as a child, but it seemed like I was pre-destined to put on weight. It's Wednesday, December 31, 2008, 11:55 pm and I'm on my knees at church praying to God. I asked him to give me strength to start back working out again. See, a lot has changed since I was a young boy with aspirations to get in shape. I am married with two kids, have a career and I am musician.

My strength and conditioning habits went south after a freak workout injury in 2003. From that point, I managed to balloon from a fit and trim 185 to 274 lbs.   I knew I had to do something!   I was falling into the same trap that many of my family members did before.   I was afraid I was going to get diabetes or something, I needed to act fast.

Well, I started working out vigorously and changed my eating habits.   In three months, I went from 274 lbs. to 225 lbs.   It was the beginning of April and I was looking and feeling good.   While I was still 40 lbs. away from my goal of 185 lbs., I was still healthy and running again.   However, as I got further into April, something changed.   I started getting tired in the middle of workouts I could normally complete with ease.

On April 10th, I weighed myself and noticed I actually was gaining weight.   I was no longer 225 lbs. I was 240 lbs.!   "What the heck is going on?" I hadn't changed my eating habits and I definitely shouldn't be gaining weight.   Another week passed. I weighed myself the following Friday. I had ballooned to 265 lbs. and I noticed massive swelling in my ankles. Something was definitely wrong!   I called my wife and we scheduled a Doctor's appointment for that following Monday.

Friday, April 24th, 2009, I went to my primary care physician to see what was going on.   At this point, my weight had ballooned to 274 lbs. "I'm confused!" I told the Doctor.   I haven't done anything different. I am working out, eating clean, but I'm gaining massive amounts of weight in very little time frames.   The Doctor informed me that the weight gain was due to the swelling of fluid that he obviously noticed in my legs. I actually had massive swelling all over my body!

The Doctor ran some preliminary tests and couldn't find anything! At the time, my blood pressure was 112/70. I didn't have high blood pressure or diabetes. The Doctor actually said, "You are the healthy fat guy I know!" He told me the swelling could come from HIV, Lupus, Thyroid issues, etc. So, he performed more blood work and urine samples and sent me on my merry way. He told me he'd call me if he saw something from my blood work that stood out.

Well, before I could get home, the Doctor's office called me. It wasn't my blood work that worried them because it hadn't got back yet, it was my urinalysis! The test came back and I had 13 grams of protein in my urine. A healthy human being is only supposed to have .016 grams of protein in their urine at most. That's a problem! The Doctor scheduled for me to get more blood work over the weekend and see a Kidney Doctor on Monday.

I arrived at the Doctor's office on Monday to meet this really old guy, who was more vertically challenged than me. I noticed right out that he had hearing issues. No, it wasn't the two hearing aids he wore; it was the fact that he made me repeat myself several times. Nonetheless, he had already reviewed my case and told me he had some preliminary diagnoses. Well, if you remember, I had taken an HIV test, so now I'm worried. I certainly didn't do anything to contract the disease, but I was afraid my life was getting ready to change drastically.

Well, this guy kept asking me questions and stalling me out until I literally screamed and yelled at him. Finally, he told me that I could have one or two things; Focal Sclerosis or something called Minimal Change Disease. See, I knew what Focal Sclerosis was, but I had no clue what Minimal Change Disease (or MCD for short) was. He scheduled me for a kidney biopsy on Thursday, April 30th.

I made it through the biopsy (after quite an event in the hospital) and I basically had to wait for the results. I have never been so nervous in my life! I know I have something, but it is between having a disease that may cause me to need a kidney transplant or some unknown disease the Doctor refuses to tell me about. Well, on May 5, 2009, I found out I had Minimal Change Disease (MCD).

MCD has its ups and downs, but the biggest problem was being on all of the meds and also losing all my strength whatsoever. My condition was progressing worst. So, I tried to get my strength back by working out. However, working out made my condition worst. On June 25th, the Doctor wrote me a letter and advised me to stop working out until further notice. Well, not working out caused me to remain at 274 lbs. after gaining the weight due to fluid, then losing it due to meds, then gaining it back (due to meds and lack of exercise).

Well, time passed with me feeling miserable and out of shape. It had to be around November of 2010. So, I went over to my Uncle's to get a haircut. Guess who I saw over there, Leon Welch! I told him about my problem and what the Doctor told me. I asked him (again); "Can you help me?" The reluctance in his face looked all too familiar! Thank God, he relented! We started working out December 2010 and as of right now, I haven't stop since! It seemed like as soon as I got back with Leon, not only did my condition improve, but I was back to losing weight and feeling great. From December 2010 until now, I've lost over 70 lbs. and I'm still keeping it off. I'm stronger than I ever been and I feel amazing! Leon Welch showed me how to breathe at a time when I thought all was lost.

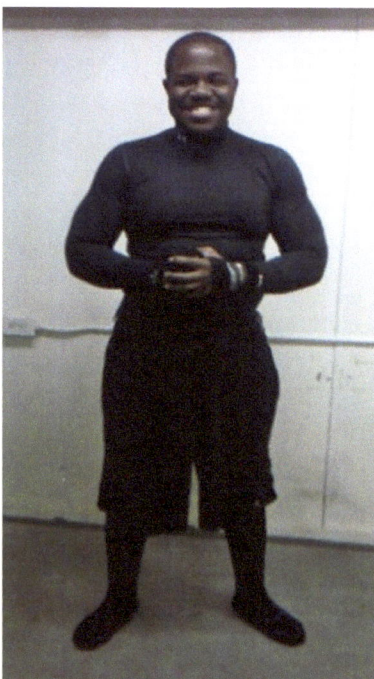

"I am now helping others!"

Things I do to Help Me Breathe

I thank Jerome for believing in me and him. He inspired me to write this book so that others could prosper and be in good health. Listed below are some guidelines that I challenge myself to live by:

Nutrition

- Drink water, less soda.
- Eat Oatmeal.
- Choose from a variety of fruits.
- Try some yogurt, low fat cheese, lactaid milk and lactose free ice cream. I'm Lactose intolerant!
- Try some Wheat or Whole Grain Bread.
- Eat chicken, fish, turkey, (sparingly eat red or fried meats- try bake, grill or broiled).
- Peanut butter and jelly.
- Eat vegetables frozen or fresh- dark green, yellow, orange, etc.
- I limit fried, salted and combination foods.
- Try unsalted cashews/almonds.
- Sweets – I try to eat sparingly, mainly at lunch time or occasionally.
- Coffee or tea- ½ cup, I use nondairy creamer/little sugar or unsweet.

- Sport waters- hour before after exercise.
- *I eat most of my starches (breads, cereals, rice, pasta ,etc.) at breakfast and lunch and between those meals
- Some foods may induce an asthma attack so know your food triggers. *Get tested for food   allergies.
- Choose low fat food sources and read food labels for ingredients and serving sizes
- Make an appointment to see a Registered Dietitian – find out how many calories you need daily and receive your individualized meal plan which may help you maintain, lose or gain weight, whatever your nutritional needs are.
- Consult with your Doctor before taking any form of nutritional drinks or supplements!

Fitness

- I keep my fast acting inhaler with me at all times.
- I walked a mile before I jogged it.
- I try to walk or jog for at least 150 minutes a week.
- I prefer walking or jogging in the evening.
- I will exercise indoors if it's too cold or hot outside.
- I choose activities that I like to participate in.
- I purchased running shoes that reduce the foot and leg pain I experienced while running outdoors on hard pavement.
- I weight train 2 to 3 times a week. I target the 9 major muscle groups. Two exercises to three exercises per muscle anywhere from 6 reps to 20 reps, 3 to 4 sets.
- Try to get up to 8 hours of sleep to recuperate from working all day and exercising.
- Consult with your Doctor before starting an exercise program.
- Find you a personal trainer that can get you in the right direction.
- Find someone with like-minded goals to exercise with you.

Wellness

- Think positive! You are what you think.
- Crawl before you walk. Start off slow. It's a lifestyle, not a quick fix.
- Take time out your day to relax.
- Get a massage.
- Everything you do for you should be a benefit.
- Remove anything that causes you stress or serves as an obstacle to achieving your goals!
- Seek counseling services if you feel like giving up.
- Join a support group that can help you get started. Church, community outreach center, local recreation centers, fitness center, etc.
- Laugh.
- Make short and long term goals. Once achieved, help others!

Conclusion

When I am not having problems with Asthma or Allergies, I take advantage of this moment. I take things one day at a time. My battle is within. Sometimes it's hard for me to gather up strength to eat right and exercise especially when I get ill. I have experienced two severe Asthma attacks in my life, one a year ago. My fiancé, my sunshine, the love of my life, saved my life. She brought me to the Emergency Room right on time. Cecilia Aguirre, I thank you for your love, patience, and being my support system. I could not have completed this book without you.

www.ingramcontent.com/pod-product-compliance
Lightning Source LLC
Chambersburg PA
CBHW041222270326
41933CB00001B/14